A Doctor In A Patient's Body:

Dreaming Big With Sickle Cell Disease And
Chronic Pain.

Simone Eastman Uwan M.D.

Praises for "A Doctor In A Patient's Body":

"A Doctor In a Patient's Body not only gives hard to come by, valuable information and life experiences on living with Sickle Cell disease, but it is also inspirational and aspirational. Simone takes the reader on the ride of a Sickle Cell warrior and drops gold nuggets along the way. You won't regret giving it a read." **~ Gabrielle Davis, Founder of Lupus Sistas and Lupus Patient Advocate.**

"An insightful account about a thoughtful and courageous physician living with Sickle Cell Disease. Her illness does not subdue her. She is a one of a kind Sickle Cell warrior, and a seasoned advocate." **~Brenda James, M.D. General Pediatrician, San Juan Health Partners Pediatrics.**

"I believe this book is a must read for anyone in chronic pain and particularly those who suffer from Sickle Cell disease. As a physician myself it serves as a painful reminder of how far short we fall in truly caring for our patients' deepest needs." **~Dr. Bill Byrd, Family Medicine physician at Family Physicians Group in Longwood Florida.**

"An inspirational and motivational account of "thriving" with Sickle Cell disease. This book shows by example that people with chronic pain and a lifelong disease can still make a powerful impact if they follow their calling. This book is a must read for all Sickle Cell patients, their family, friends and the medical providers caring for them." **~Allan Platt, PA-C, MMSc, DFAAPA, Asst. Professor, Dir. of Admissions Physician Assistant Program, Emory University School of Medicine.**

"Truly inspirational... An amazing journey through rough times but with a bright outcome. A beacon for the many lost in a fog of stereotypes. I believe healthcare providers who read this book will have their perspective on Sickle Cell patients changed for the better." **~Pierre Fotso M.D., Assoc. Director of Inpatient Medicine, Orlando Regional Medical Center**

"Thorough a series of short stories, Dr. Simone Uwan manages to paint a colorful and detailed perspective on what it is like to live with a chronic illness. She allows you to feel the self-doubt, reactions of others, and challenges in her journey. You also become witness to the faith, resilience, and optimism that Simone has nurtured in her life that has clearly led her to thrive with Sickle Cell disease." **~Laura Salazar MD, AAHIVS Chair, Department of Internal Medicine, Hoag Medical Group**

Foreword

I'm excited to write this foreword for Dr. Simone Eastman Uwan. Simone and I met at Stanford University School of Medicine. What started out as a colleague friendship, quickly became a lifelong family relationship enduring all these years later. From study sessions to game nights with friends, weddings, and graduations, Simone has extraordinary personality that makes you want to spend time with her. Simone and her husband Aniekan have a special bond and a distinct place in our hearts with us watching our children grow up, celebrating our milestones, and sympathizing with our losses. Simone and I can talk deeply, and

Simone has had quite a life battling Sickle Cell disease. She does most things we do, in pain, yet she is no victim. People want to be around her because she gives generously of herself. She does not hesitate to say, "I love you!" She also does not hesitate to pray, for everything! She has a whole-hearted kind of faith. You would forget that she is struggling if not for her oxygen tank and cane. I admire Simone for her unwavering faith and kindness. She has experienced the unimaginable at times and no matter what is always finding the positive and being a beacon of light.

What she has accomplished with her Sickle Cell disease is nothing short of amazing and speaks volumes about her character of perseverance and forgiveness. She has lived with Sickle Cell disease as both the patient and the doctor, and she is the first doctor I know to write personally about this disease. This alone is an accomplishment! Her books-because there will be others-will inspire and motivate people with Sickle Cell disease, influence people who care for people with Sickle Cell disease, and encourage others dealing with challenges in life. May the world be forever changed by her stories.

Congratulations Dr. Simone Eastman Uwan on publishing your first book!

~ Stacey Jolly M.D., Stanford University School of Medicine alumna

Acknowledgements

For my mom Olivia: kudos to that brave young woman who yielded to God so He could bring me into the world. Kudos to the single mom who raised us. I am forever grateful. I love you!

For my husband Aniekan, my superman and soulmate. I'm grateful you chose to make me your "chocolate drop". Thank you for loving me enough to walk this journey with me and for making it your daily mission to make me laugh. I am amazed that you love me like a new bride after 21 years.

To my sister, Natasha; how I love you! God blessed me with you for a little sister. Your heart of kindness and compassion and sheer love for me is quite rare. I'm a lucky big sister indeed!

I also want to especially thank Annette Peinado, Dr. Brenda James, Dr. Laura Salazar and Dr. Stacey Jolly for your support in making this book happen! Thank you also for being such a special part of my journey.

Lastly, thank you to my friend of decades Angela Abrahams-Gibson for guiding me to the finish line with this book. You were the angel I prayed for.

And to the MANY beautiful people that have been the wind beneath my wings, I thank you too! I live because you love.

Table of Contents

PART III

Prologue

To write this book has been nothing short of a divine calling. I am reluctant to say that at the time I was told to write this book, I decided I liked what I was already doing, and viewed the calling like a suggestion. I was working as a Family Practice Doctor and enjoying giving back to underserved patients.

But I was struggling to juggle my life as somebody's daughter, wife, sister and friend with being a physician and a very high-maintenance patient. I always felt like I was walking a tightrope. One false move, and the cookie would crumble.

I used to volunteer at a week-long Sickle Cell summer camp. I did this for a few years, volunteering as one of their many doctors to care for the children. But it became not so fun when one year I spent half the time curled up on a bed in the infirmary myself! What a sight! So, I "ran away" by deciding not to return to the camp that following year.

I was part of an online support group, also for many years. This community really helped me to feel included and understood with my Sickle Cell disease. When I became a doctor, I started answering medical questions for the group. However, there came a time when the medical questions came fast and furious, and I could not respond to them quickly enough. It only revealed my limitations and left some people with unanswered questions and hurt feelings. I was failing the very community that was so dear to me.

At the very same time, I was failing yet another group; my local Sickle Cell chapter right here in Orlando. I started out with great intentions too! But they were across town. Unbeknownst to everyone, I was having flares of pain from driving and was needing to be chauffeured even to work. So, I ran away by deciding to pull back from both groups and concentrate on juggling life as a patient and a doctor instead.

So why would I be tapped to do this assignment? What I do know is that it has become apparent that I was only meant to have one season of my life at a time. I also know that the last decade of life has changed much of the way I think about things. As I age I wonder what my legacy would be, and I ask myself where I would like to spend the next years of my life. And I would like to pass on whatever I can to others, however big or small, if it can be of any help.

So God in his amazing patience, mercy and love has helped me to stop running like Jonah in the Bible. And now, it is time to get to work.

I choose to write my first book on Sickle Cell disease, about my journey through college. It was during these years that I became gravely ill and got my diagnosis, something that would forever change my life and the lives of my loved ones. It represents my formative years with Sickle Cell and reveals a lot about the struggles I went through to make it through college, while also trying to reaffirm my worth. But it also tells of my refusal to give up and how I found some unconventional ways of coping, that I use even now. For this reason, I believe everyone can still learn something from reading this book. I will share my journey with you in the hopes that you can find both commonality and inspiration to blaze your own trail. *THAT* is my intention; that you discover all the areas that you can grow, and you go for it!

4

PART I

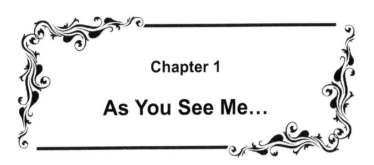

Chapter 1

As You See Me...

Today there is so much I'm grateful for that I have accomplished. At age 13 I immigrated to the United States from Guyana, South America, and for the first year lived with my grandmother on Lewis Avenue in Brooklyn, New York. I went to Sarah Garnet Junior High School, about five blocks from my residence, and was there for one year before starting at Clara Barton High School.

I excelled in high school and graduated ranking 3rd in a class of 538 graduating students. I received several scholarships to attend Barnard College, Columbia University in New York City, where I studied biology and was a pre-medical student. While I was a believer in Christ prior to this point, I seriously studied the bible and got baptized at the start of my freshman year of college. I majored in Biology and pre-medical studies there at Columbia University.

After graduating, I moved to California where I did research for one year at UCLA while applying to medical school. I was granted admission to Stanford University School of Medicine, one of the top medical schools in the United States. During medical school I received both a Medical Scholar Award and a Pfeiffer Scholar Award for medical research I did. I was featured in several Stanford Medical magazines for my research. I also contributed my personal written story to a non-fiction book called "What I Learned In Medical School; Personal Stories of Young Doctors". In 1997, soon after my second year of medical school, and after two years of dating, I was married to my superman, Aniekan. We recently celebrated 21 years of marriage.

Chapter 1~ As You See Me...

I graduated medical school and was accepted to a Stanford-affiliated Family Practice Residency program, where I did specialized training in Family Medicine. Upon completion I became Board Certified in Family Medicine and soon after was employed as a Family Practice physician. I cared for patients of all ages by providing prenatal care, and seeing pediatric, adolescent and adult patients, including reproductive age women and geriatric care. And I loved it all.

All this sounds wonderful right? You are probably saying, "Sign me up! I would not mind trading places with you". However, while this might appear as a wonderful picture to many, it was not a rosy journey by any means. In fact, there were many times that I almost walked away.

What I have not yet shared with you is that I am a Sickle Cell warrior. I say warrior because my journey for the most part has been nothing short of a fight for my life. So let me roll back the curtains and show you what really happened. I will share my journey with you. That includes my lowest lows, my greatest joys, and my lessons learned along the way. I will also show you how I was able to accomplish my goals, in the hopes that by the end of the time we have spent together, I will have inspired you to accomplish yours too. Where do I begin? I guess my point of breakdown that lead to breakthrough is as good a place as any to begin. Let's start with an introduction to Sickle Cell disease, both for you and for me. Let's start with my diagnosis.

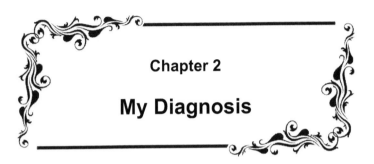

Chapter 2

My Diagnosis

Today what I share with you I am writing down for the first time. I don't talk about this part of my life much, because truthfully it is all still a blur, with many of the details having been provided to me afterwards. I've had to grow into my understanding of some parts as well, both medically and spiritually.

Earlier in the year of 1990, during the second semester of my sophomore year of college, I started having intense abdominal pains. There were a couple of times that I laid down for almost half a day and could not get up from the floor of my dormitory. I have this affinity for floors because usually my pain feels so intense and hot that I almost want to put that part of my body against a cool surface. And while I had been sick like this before, it had been a long time that it had gotten to this extent.

Our Student Health Services department did my bloodwork and told me that I had the "Sickle Cell trait" and should be concerned about getting married to someone else with a Sickle Cell trait because it could give the disease to my children. And that was that. As far as I knew I was good. Later as my pain worsened, and as I kept passing out at church and different places, I was given a million different diagnoses. One doctor at St. Luke Hospital told me that maybe my fainting was because I was "getting slain in the spirit"! She said our black churches were very passionate during worship. She actually said that! I looked at my friend that came with me from church. Just because the two of us were people of color she assumed that we went to a black church. And nothing could be further from the truth. But that was my diagnosis that day. My pain and loss of consciousness was as a result of my passionate worship at church.

Later I would be told by Student Health Services that my constant abdominal pains were likely "trapped gas." Gas got new respect from me that day, because the pain I felt left me almost lifeless by the end of each episode. Finally, the same doctors encouraged that I get an abdominal ultrasound, which unfortunately showed a couple of ovarian cysts. I say unfortunately because this turned out to be an incidental finding, not the real reason for my pains at all. But because of this I was started on birth control pills to manage the cysts. That turned out to be the single worst thing that could have been done because unfortunately my undiagnosed Sickle Cell disease was already pre-disposing me to clotting problems, and birth control pills could certainly cause a clot.

It was late August 1990. I was returning from Canada where I was visiting relatives with my mother. I returned to campus and went to take a nap but woke up shortly after feeling like my lungs were on fire and falling out of my chest. I was supposed to get together with someone for a tutoring session, and true to character did not cancel the session but instead invited my friend to join me in the ER at Columbia Presbyterian Hospital to figure out why I felt like dying.

It turns out the reason I felt like dying was because I WAS dying- in bits and pieces anyway. I remember a few things about my ER experience that day. As soon as they checked my temperature and realized that I was running a very high fever, and saw that my EKG was abnormal, they put me on a gurney likely to make sure that I would not collapse. And that was it; lights out.

The next time my eyes opened was several days later, at around 4 AM in the morning. I was surrounded by a team of doctors in the ICU, all looking at me and talking to each other. I heard whispers of "welcome back" and "so glad you're awake", all shrouded in tones of concern. Soon after someone left to get my mom, who seemed to have been living there, camped out with friends and family. I could not talk to anyone because a machine had been breathing for me during this time. The tubes were still in my mouth and down my throat, with tape anchoring the outside part of the tubing to my face.

This felt familiar. This felt like 1982 with my first major hospitalization where I almost died. Except once again my life was spared. I looked directly across from me to see a huge collage made for me. Seeing the direction of my gaze, my mom who was now present, and puffy with tears of joy, explained that this was a collage made by all my friends from my campus ministry. I read signs of "get well soon" and "we love you" with tons of pictures of me and my friends taken together in various places. There were scriptures written, with every imaginable encouragement. And some of my friends were outside! In fact, many had refused to go home, staying long hours and keeping vigil, praying, doing their homework in the waiting rooms, hallways and stairways. They took turns seeing me since only two were allowed in the ICU room at a time. They would pray over me and return to the outside waiting rooms to talk with and comfort my family members. Apparently, they had crowded out the living spaces, causing the nurses and doctors to ask if I was an unrecognized celebrity of some sort.

Chapter 2~ My Diagnosis

Turns out I was just one "sister" out of many sisters and brothers from our campus ministry. We were like a team. And we had spent the last two years studying in school and hanging out together. We met as a group on Wednesday for midweek bible studies, Friday for special campus devotionals/Game nights, and Sunday for services. We had gotten close and they were not about to leave me behind. And that was their way of showing it. They were going to wait and pray until I woke up.

I had been unconscious for almost a week. Time had gone by while I laid sleeping. And yet it felt like time had stood still. All I wanted to do was relay a message, but I was still not breathing on my own. However, I was obviously improving because I had slowly started bucking the vent, a term used when people are getting stronger and wanting to breathe on their own.

Chapter 2~ My Diagnosis

So much happened that's hard to say or write, in part because I STILL do not understand it all. But the girl who woke up in that ICU was in some way a different person than my friends had known.

The girl who woke up asked for a pen and paper to scrawl:

"I SAW GOD" and later "HEAVEN IS REAL."

One of the things I don't understand to this day is how to explain where I was during the time I was on life support. Had I actually died? Was I just teetering on the brink, when God showed up? Why would He hang out with ME? Wasn't He busy dealing with the world, the prayers of humanity, world wars and such?

And how was I able to hear people who were in the ICU at my bedside?

At one point some of the campus ministry staff came by to encourage my family. As they stood over my ICU bed speaking with my family, I could hear them so clearly! At one point, Leslie one of the staff members visiting with her husband said, "if you can hear me, squeeze my hand." I must've just felt it happen because apparently nothing on my body moved, and after a while they agreed that I could not squeeze their hand, and that I should just rest. It did not help that the nursing staff and even a doctor kept telling people that I could not hear them. How would they know? Had they ever been here? And where is "here" anyway?! I was so frustrated! I wanted to say "but I CAN hear everything you're saying to me Leslie! And I can hear your conversation with my family too!

Because of the way time seemed to have stood still, it is difficult to determine where in the course of my unconsciousness this happened. Was it towards the beginning or the end that they came to visit? Was I just "leaving" or "returning"? I truly cannot say.

What I will never forget is hearing my mom's voice asking me to come back. She was so drained by the whole ordeal and so desperate for me to "return to her", that she pleaded to me as I laid there on that ICU bed. "Come back to me honey", she said. "If you come back I promise I will study the Bible". And on she went with her pleading and promising.

I could not believe I was hearing this from my mom! This was indeed a game changer! This was my mom who had given me quite a hard time, saying that I was giving too much time to my new-found Christianity, and that she was concerned for my grades. However, with my grades going steadily up since the first semester of my freshman year, there had not been much to work with. No jabs of "I told you so". Instead, she slowly started complementing the fact that I was more helpful and serving at home. She even became interested in meeting my friends. However, that was as far as it was going to go. No coming to church with me. That's where she drew the line. Yet here she was telling me that she would study the Bible IF I came back.

I immediately started asking God to return. It had been an amazing time. Had nothing else happened, I would have wanted to stay. But with my mother telling me this, I suddenly saw a whole world of change possible for my family, and it meant everything to me that they could one day make it to heaven. So, I begged to come back. And I remember very clearly what I was told.

"It's OK Simone, you may go back. But when you come again, make sure you bring your family with you."

And just like that, I was making my way back.

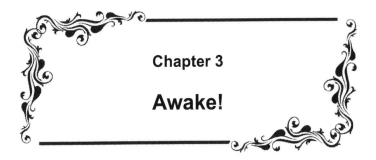

Chapter 3

Awake!

I was awake, but by no means well. I was still not out of the woods. I had barely made it back and everything was fuzzy and in pieces as I drifted in and out of sleep over the next several days.

My lung had collapsed I was told. I had suffered a massive pulmonary embolism and the entire right lower lobe had infarcted (death of lung tissue from blockage in circulation and lack of oxygen to the area). I had spiked high fevers of 105°F and above that caused damage to muscle tissue throughout my body. They had done every imaginable test on me and determined that I had something called Sickle Cell disease. Mom said that they were amazed that she did not know that this is what I had all along, because in the United States children were diagnosed at birth in all 50 states. But I had been born in Guyana, in a land with different rules, and I had fallen through the cracks.

Oh, my goodness! This is what my sick childhood had been all about! This explains the fainting episodes in school. My hospitalization at age 12 years old had caused great compromise to my lungs then too, with flooding of both sides of my lungs and serious pulmonary complications. This is what it had ALL been about; this thing called Sickle Cell disease.

It is hard to talk to someone about what happened while I slept. It was a precious experience to me; precious and private. Talking about it and watching someone trying to dissect it to make it have earthly sense seems to somehow take away the sacredness of the experience. The message I wrote on that piece of paper had circulated to the friends and family that came to visit. Later I regretted not waiting to give careful instructions on how to share that message with people. What was precious to me seemed like it had been shared in such a way that it become fantastical, almost like a freak show conversation. That was the last thing I wanted! And it was of EXTREME importance to me not to embellish the story or exaggerate my experience.

Even now, I cannot remember the sequence of things and how they unfolded once I woke up. My memory of everything that happened around me appeared in flashes.

Flash ... I'm being transfused units of blood. Flash ...a kind nurse named "Glo" (Gloria?) has me on my stomach on something that tilts my body down, feet up as she firmly beats my back with cupped palms(percussions)to drain the fluid from

Chapter 3 ~ Awake!

my chest. I'm told I have suffered an episode of what is called "Acute Chest Syndrome" which is a severe form of respiratory distress, and the leading cause of death for Sickle Cell patients. Flash...a long needle is being poked into my back to draw fluid from my lung. Flash...I've been transferred to a regular floor and I'm not handling it well at all! I am later told by my family that I "coded" and had to be rushed back to ICU. I can only remember fading away into unconsciousness as a team of doctors rushed to my bedside, slapping me and saying "wake up Simone! Stay with us! You can't do this to us!" Believe it or not, I actually remembered that.

Flash...I have no spleen anymore. Previous ultrasound had shown a spleen, but damage from Sickle Cell the past year had left its evidence. The entire organ was destroyed and was completely gone! No trace of it was left. The doctors asked me if I had ever experienced episodes of intense abdominal pain. I think back to my diagnosis of "gas pains" or being "slain in the spirit". So much for those theories.

Flash...I can't walk! The high fevers have caused muscle damage I'm told. I need to have rehabilitation therapy and learn to hold myself up and walk again. If I can't do this I can't go home. It would take over one month to get home. But as it turned out, home was the beginning of another long journey; the journey of my life with my new diagnosis of Sickle Cell disease. Unfortunately, it was a new diagnosis, but the disease had been present in my body all along. And I had plenty to show for it.

As I was being prompted in my spirit to share all this in my book, I could not help wondering what was the relevance of sharing this with people. Back then there were a few naysayers too, and this time around there will likely be more. I am also well aware that this is not a religious book. But then I remember my audience – you! You my Sickle Cell survivors and fellow pain warriors have probably had many of these hospitalizations where you fought for life as you danced on the edge of earth and heaven. And when you opened your eyes, if you tried to tell that story, people stared at you with glazed over eyes as they did with me. And maybe you decided it was better left unsaid.

I was once at a huge congregational service in San Francisco where a little boy with Sickle Cell disease shared that he "died and met God and talked with Him". I could hear the muttering in the congregation even as he continued to share. Probably most people did not hear anything past that sentence. But I sat on my chair fixated on the child, because it was the first time someone had shared a part of my story. And I knew he was telling the truth!

Maybe I am meant to validate your story. Maybe you dissected it and tried to make it have earthly sense and when it didn't, you threw it away. Or maybe you were still holding it in your heart as a precious experience that you could never share. Whatever it is, I am supposed to share with you that you are not alone.

A lot happened to my body as you can imagine. The other parts of my admission are difficult to share as well. But again, I'm sharing the whole process of what happened, because many of you I'm sure can relate to things falling apart while you watch. My hope is that if you saw yourself in any part of my story, you will begin to see that my successes can be yours too.

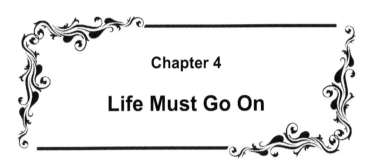

Chapter 4

Life Must Go On

The year that followed was spent at home recuperating. It was a year filled with bi-monthly blood exchange transfusions (removal of my sickled red blood cells and replacement with donated red blood cells) to prevent further damage to my severely compromised lungs. I worked on getting my physical strength back and understanding what my daily life was going to be like as a result of the damage my body had endured to this point.

Until now, I had battled Sickle Cell disease without any intervention, treatment or pain management. There was great damage to my nerves and tissues, which was starting to manifest in chronic pain that needed management. In many ways it was a relief to have a diagnosis, because now I could have some sort of therapy. That started with a pain management specialist and a Pulmonologist besides my Hematologist and Primary Care Physician.

It was a rough year, but I was determined to figure out how to return to school and continue my studies. To process all that was changing, I wrote about my experiences as I went. There were many pain-filled days where I was fated to bond with my bed. In an effort to turn my lemons into lemonade, lemon drops and lemon chess pie, I used these times to write. As I returned to school and learned how to navigate my way through being a pre-medical student, and even as I battled beyond college, my bed was a constant place of writing.

Many of the reflective pieces I wrote I will share with you in this book, as they will shed light and illuminate a path that hopefully you can follow when the time comes. They are NOT chronological, but a collection of stories placed in an order I felt was best. Please remember this as you read! I call my writings "Bedtime Stories with Doctor Simone Uwan", and appropriately so, as they are stories of my life, written with my struggling hands as I wrote in pain from my bed.

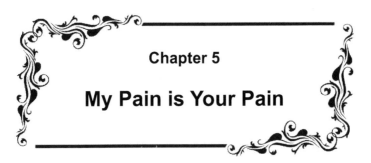

Chapter 5

My Pain is Your Pain

I want to share with you what my life with Sickle Cell disease has been like, so that you are comfortable with knowing that to some extent, I understand and feel your pain too. I know that no two Sickle Cell individuals will present the same, but we will recognize the symptoms when we hear about it. There are certain commonalities that reassure us we are dealing with the same disease.

My Sickle Cell pain symptoms have many components. There's burning, there is aching, and many times there are random stabbing pains that would make me jump in the middle of a sentence, scaring many of my friends and family. The pain is usually in my upper chest, mid-back, forearms and bilateral lower legs including my knees. Those places are consistent. Other times I can have neck, abdominal and thigh pain.

Sometimes I have had chest pain with left arm or leg numbness and tingling and went so many times to the ER thinking I had a heart attack or stroke (both of which I have had before). Other times it has been severe headaches lasting for a day or so. The intensity of pain on an average day when I am well is about a 3 to 4 out of 10 on a chronic morphine regimen. About 4 to 5 days a week it is between 4 and 7 out of 10 at random times of the day, depending on where I am (cold) or what I'm doing (exertion).

About once per month my Sickle Cell crisis pain is 8 to 10 out of 10, usually the week preceding and the week of my menstrual cycle. In the past it has landed me in the hospital almost every month until I figured out some ways to lessen the severity to where I could suffer through it at home with morphine and other medications and supplements, along with home oxygen and aggressive hydration. This is what I do at home now for most of my moderate Sickle Cell crises.

The things that cause me to experience Sickle Cell pain episodes include any exertion like exercising that causes oxygen depletion and ischemia, or tissue damage. Walking long distances or standing too long does the same thing. Driving has progressively caused localized pain flares in my forearms and legs presumed to be from muscle fatigue, so that my driving has become very limited. I first noticed this when I could no longer drive myself to work. I would arrive at work in a Sickle Cell crisis, even before my clinic day had started! I had to get a driver to drop me off and pick me up so as to maximize my energy and minimize my pain.

Chapter 5~My Pain is Your Pain

Often my self care became compromised. I would have someone braid my hair once per month to prevent triggering a Sickle Cell pain episode in my fingers with frequent combing of my hair, and to prevent using my aching right shoulder which I had been told needed surgery due to tendon ruptures. I would take showers about 4 times a week to have energy left for other things on days when I did not take a shower. In between, I used bath wipes. I can dress myself fairly well and I use a sock aid to put on my socks and sit down to put on my underwear and slacks.

For housecleaning, we usually pay or ask someone we know well once a month to do a deep housecleaning and then try to maintain by tidying up in between. I can do light tidying up fairly well. I do a little at a time when I'm doing fine so I don't fatigue much. But laundry was too hard for me. It always seemed to trigger a Sickle Cell flare, so I did not do laundry for years. These days I seem to be able to do a little more.

For shopping, on very good days, maybe about once every 2 months, I try going to a store to get clothing or things I may not want my husband to buy. Otherwise he does all the food shopping. Usually food shopping is exhausting. The stores are way too cold and trigger a painful episode within minutes of walking through the doors of the supermarket. I once had to be taken home by a stranger after setting out to the store because I got sick very suddenly and things unfolded rather quickly in the store, so I try not to put myself in danger. I'm so glad that stranger was a good soul, because I was completely vulnerable.

I love being social but I'm severely restricted. Most places outside my house are "danger zones" either because of temperatures that are too cold, or risk of exertion from walking or standing too long. Because of using the cane and not being able to walk fast with my prosthetic restrained type hip and restricted motion, I tend to wear out and stop many times in the span of one block.

My friends often visit me at home and will take the time to unwind about what is going on in their lives, sometimes asking my input about things. Or they might watch movies with me, and often will come lay down with me when I'm sick and talk with me right there. At other times I love writing poetry, reading, or watching a movie by myself and at my own pace, usually when I'm not well and can't move anyway. If I go out, it is to another person's home who can accommodate my temperature needs. Thankfully, many of my friends happily do this for me, and for this I'm very grateful.

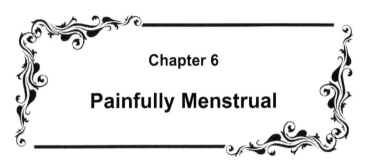

Chapter 6

Painfully Menstrual

For as far back as I can remember, each time I would get to the part of the month that I would have a menstrual cycle, there would be drama. It started a week before my cycle with a sense of feeling flushed and clammy yet cold in my whole body, like I had experienced a sharp change in the quantity of some hormone, probably a drop in either estrogen or progesterone. I say likely this because these are the two hormones in your menstrual cycle that drop right before menstruation. I would then proceed to have what I have always considered to be an associated Sickle Cell crisis with lower back pain, out of this world leg pains, and anterior chest wall pain.

Chapter 6~Painfully Menstrual

Within hours of actually having my flow start, I would have uterine cramping so hard that it felt like I was about to deliver a baby. Often it would wake me up out of my sleep. My lower back and waist would hurt so badly, along with a throbbing pain that radiated from my abdomen down into my pelvis, and out my vagina. I would curl up into a fetal position, grateful for the bathroom's tiled floor and the coolness it provided against my flushed and sweating body. I would feel like I was going to vomit at the same time. My mouth would spring salty water.

I finally figured out that if I used magnesium in large quantities within days leading up to the start of my cycle, it greatly minimized these episodes. Coupling that with substantial doses of calcium in a holistic preparation of essential minerals and vitamins significantly reduced the cramping episodes at the beginning of each cycle.

Chapter 6~Painfully Menstrual

But it took a long time to figure that out. So, when an episode started I would just reach for ibuprofen 200 mg tablets and take four of them, for a total of 800 mg, which is the prescription strength. It did help a little. Then I would lay there until the cramping episode was over. It seemed like forever, but it would take about an hour or so. Once I started anticoagulation therapy, I was told I could no longer use ibuprofen, for risk of bleeding out. It was truly dramatic.

The rest of the week was a blur of pain from the Sickle Cell crisis that ensued. For most of it I was literally bedridden, with life passing by in a haze of pain. My goals for those days was to brush my teeth, get my body cleaned up somehow, and get something to eat. I made plans to cook and store food for me and my husband prior to that week most times, but once in a while I was taken off guard and needed some extra help getting food to eat.

Chapter 6~Painfully Menstrual

The intensity of my menstrual cycle with triggered Sickle Cell crisis would range from me being hospitalized and needing a blood transfusion and pain management, to outpatient IV hydration at the infusion center of my Hematologist and then rest with pain management at home. Even though staying at home and using only outpatient infusion of IV fluids was not optimal, I always felt better being in my own bed, not being attached to the machines like in the hospital, and not having nurses assume that I was a drug seeker versus being in excruciating pain. If only to spare me that, this was way better.

In my earlier years I tried using the Depo-Provera injection, a form of birth control that did not have estrogen like the regular birth controls pills, because this would put me at risk for blood clots. Over time however, the "Depo shot" caused thinning of my bones which finally led to osteoporosis. I'm grateful that I was able to find a holistic healthcare provider that started a treatment which slowly reversed my osteoporosis back to normal bone. My Primary Care doctor and Endocrinologist were shocked, because this did not happen much in conventional medicine.

Alas though, we were never able to declare victory over my menstrual cycles. When my holistic practitioner suddenly (and sadly) passed away, my situation slowly returned to the monthly bane of my existence, save for the comfort provided by magnesium and calcium. Often the only rescue was a blood transfusion, and for many years this was my lot every four weeks. Regardless of what was going on in my life, life came to a standstill. I-needed-blood.

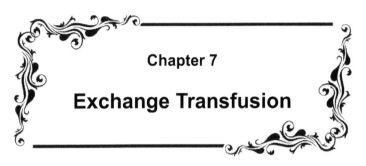

Chapter 7

Exchange Transfusion

So basically, my seriously mutated red blood cells decided to play hooky and not do their job. And it was a simple "delivery man/ paper route" job. No big deal. They just pick up a bulk of oxygen from the central station at Mrs. Lungs, and make the deliveries, distributing around the neighborhood (body) so that everyone has some oxygen to use for the day. But my blood cells had decided that they were too bent out of shape from all the stresses of life, and they decided to call in sick.

This unfortunately often left ME unable to show up for life. So, I needed full body blood exchange transfusions-about 4 to 5 units of blood- to do the

Chapter 7 ~ Exchange Transfusion

job that I was already paying(nourishing) my red blood cells to do. Except my red cells were wasting my energy growing themselves plump, and not giving me back much in return. At least that's what I thought back then. Instead, I lived with the help of people's blood.

But nothing could prepare me for this one experience I was about to have. It was soon after I had been diagnosed, and I had finally been discharged from the hospital. After being there for a month and experiencing too many life altering events to count, I was happy to be home. I was 19 years old and learning to walk again, but my right lower lobe of my lung had been wrecked by extensive sickling. My body needed a "time out" from these sickling episodes so it could heal.

So, my mom would take me to the transfusion center where I would receive full body exchange

Chapter 7 ~ Exchange Transfusion

transfusions every three weeks. They would take out small amounts of my blood at a time, separate out my red blood cells and provide me with some healthy and durable ones that would last longer, closer to their usual life span of one hundred and twenty days. This was definitely an upgrade from my red blood cells with their lifespan of twenty to thirty days, and afterwards I felt like superwoman!

But today, for whatever reason, I was not passing out all over the place during the exchange transfusion, which had become my Modus Operandi. No stopping the procedure to tilt my recliner chair head down, no smelling salts, and no slapping me in the face to bring me back to consciousness while my mom watched helplessly. No, today I was rather calm, observing each step of the process. The cherry red blood flowed from my right arm through a needle in my veins and

Chapter 7 ~ Exchange Transfusion

into a tubing, which then coiled through a circular pumping device that rotated, causing my blood to be emptied into a receiving bag as the tube ended. At the same time, at the very same rate, the burgundy blood on the I.V pole flowed from a donor bag down a connecting tube and through the needle into my left arm veins. So the needle in my right arm and the needle in my left arm had blood coming and going at equal rate.

I was admiring my newly acquired blood when I happened to look up and see the nurse disconnecting a full bag of my red blood cells. It looked great in the bag! As matter of fact, it resembled the donor bag on my right. And just as I wondering what she would do with it, where she would send it, and what great science research was going to be done with it, she, without even stopping the chatter with her other nurse friends, raised her hand and tossed my blood into a red trash bag, located in a red trash can marked HAZARDOUS WASTE on the outside.

I wished I had never seen that.

That was one day I wished *I really had* passed out! It felt like she had thrown *ME* into the trash. It was the first time that I realized how sacred blood had become to me. After all, it sustained my *life*. To throw it away felt like something sacred became profane. That was so hard for me to see.

No matter though. I still walked out of Columbia-Presbyterian Blood Transfusion Center feeling like superwoman, full of the right stuff! The right kind of somebody's blood that was letting me live. And I wanted to be conscious and live the heck out of that blood for the next three weeks. And the blood three weeks after that, and after that. So I did!

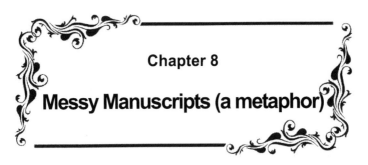

Chapter 8

Messy Manuscripts (a metaphor)

I am walking with a manuscript. It is typewritten single spaced, a beautiful story unfolding. But without warning something or someone shoves me from behind, and to my alarm my arms are too weak to hold on to the pages of the manuscript. So down I go falling to my belly.

Where are those pages? They are everywhere! Scattered everywhere! And there are so many pieces of precious paper. I slowly lift myself up, dust myself off, and bend over to pick up the pages. People pass by in a hurry and some of them step on the pages of my manuscript. They don't mean to, but everything is everywhere, and in their path and they have to get to their destination. In the meantime, I smile an apology that cannot make it through my lips. I feel ashamed that I have inconvenienced everyone going everywhere. I try to pick up the pieces as quickly as possible out of people's path, hoping I could recover all the pages. Some are damaged. Some have footprints, and some have holes where the spiked heels of fancy shoes poked through the pages. All are out of order. But thankfully all are there.

I stand up still weak from the impact of the fall, and with a smile on my face, hoping that no one really understands the depth of what just happened. Thankfully, everyone is busy, and hardly noticed that I was just knocked over. Or maybe some noticed but would rather not talk about it. I am glad, because if they had stopped long enough to ask, they would know that this is the third time this month that I've been knocked over. They would notice that I get knocked over many many times, and the consequences are visible on different parts of my body. There are cuts too deep for just a Band-Aid. Some might see that I'm still bleeding from the last fall. Many of the old wounds have not healed.

I gather my many pages, all out of sequence. As people continue to pass by, at least for the ones I know, I continue the conversations as though nothing had happened just moments ago. I ask them, "How are you? How is your mom? How is your little one?". I act as though nothing was out of the ordinary, all while I try to put the pieces of my story back together. And they take their time and tell me all about their lives, all while the cuts bleed down my legs and into my shoes.

I wish I could tell you differently. I wish I could tell you that this manuscript is a book that I could put on a shelf, so that the next time I fell things would be easier. But this my friend, is not a story of fiction. I am Simone, and this manuscript is a metaphor, for my life.

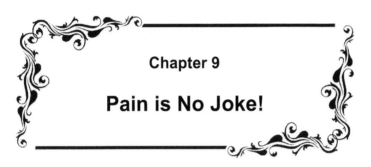

Chapter 9

Pain is No Joke!

Have you ever hurt so much, that you became skewed in your thinking? I hurt so much that I started to believe I was just going through meaningless suffering, and I wanted to give up. And by that, I mean permanently. Pain skewed my thinking and made me waver.

One summer, my pain was so out of control in both my body and my heart that I thought it best if I were not here on earth anymore. I was in an emotional roller coaster about school and how my life had been put on pause. I felt like I was free falling. To make matters worse, there was an upset I was overcoming in a friendship, with feelings of betrayal running high. In times like those, the last thing you need is to have a Sickle Cell crisis that would not seem to end. I remember watching everyone leave to enjoy the festivities of a July summer day, and on that bright and sunny day, I laid alone at home in my bed, watching the world go by and feeling like time had forgotten to include me in some of its minutes. And the pain was too much. I decided I wanted to die.

Fortunately for me, I was found by my family before irreversible damage could occur. That day for whatever reason, they had decided to come home early from wherever they had gone. When it was all over, I ended up in the emergency room getting my stomach pumped and being hospitalized for treatment.

What truly dark days those were! I thought I would never stop hurting. I hated the pain I felt in my body. I was upset and disappointed that God had not taken it away like I prayed. Over time He would teach me that it was here that He was closest to me.

I needed help and had to seek counseling starting then and intermittently for some years to wrap my mind around the fact that I still had purpose, maybe even more so! I had to learn how to breathe deeply through the pain until it subsided. I had to learn how to cry my ugly cries with tears and snot while I vented to God all that was on my heart. And I had to realize that I was not the only one with aches and upsets in life. The Christian I thought I was became very real to me.

I realized that taking care of my mental health as I dealt with my chronic illness was of absolute importance to me succeeding and living my best self. In many of our communities of color, we don't talk about needing counseling when struggling with depression triggered by chronic pain. We don't talk about mental health much at all! Yet it is so prevalent! But I realized that if I did not get the mental health care I so desperately needed, any other unresolved emotional pain I had could compound the physical pain when it started and could in a moment's notice lead to a poor or regrettable decision. Counseling was a gift I gave myself. It was a gift that reminded me that I was worth fighting for!

PART II

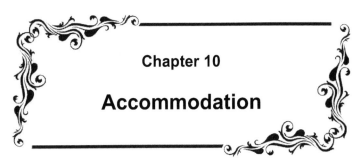

Chapter 10

Accommodation

When I returned to school, there was so much to know and do to navigate my new world. With Sickle Cell, during winter and spring breaks, I checked into the hospital to get one procedure or another, since I would finally have enough time to recuperate. Meanwhile, my classmates went to relax and regroup for winter and spring break. When it was time to study, we all studied. But when it was time for play, they played while I got "tuned up".

Many things I'm about to share with you I did not know or did not learn about until much later, but I don't want you to have to reinvent the wheel. You spend enough time being sick! So please, let me help you.

Chapter 10~ Accommodation

Again, because I wrote my recollections from my bed, they are not one continuous story, but several stories. This is not unlike our lives with this disease-lived in short intervals and interrupted often.

Here are my Bedtime Stories.

The first order of things is to register with the Office for Disability Students Services on campus, identifying yourself as someone who is in need of disability accommodation. Ask them what they would need for verification of your disability. Usually a doctor's note of your health explaining what your needs are with respect to school is required. This includes your needs during a test (extra time, a warm room, extra bathroom breaks) or even physical aids to optimize your learning in a classroom. Those sorts of things need to be listed. Do yourself a favor and draft a letter of what your needs are. Take it to your physician so they know what exactly to include in the letter-providing they agree of course.

Ask the liaison for disability affairs what other services or resources are available. Sometimes there is a "note taker" so that if you are sick and missing lectures, you can be sent a copy of the notes. Sometimes there are people available to proctor your exam in other locations. I once took the written part of an exam in the hospital because I insisted on taking it the same day as everyone else, so that when I was discharged the following day I could take the practical exam with the rest of the class. Keep in mind I was not deathly ill; I was just being admitted for a procedure that could not be postponed.

At one point, in my schooling at another campus, there was a golf cart that upon request would pick me up at an arranged time from home and take me to class. Lectures were just across campus, but it seemed to me like it was across the world because I was having sickling pains in my legs and unable to walk well. I also requested the use of an extra chair in class to raise my legs up for better circulation, and to prevent worsening a Sickle Cell flare (better known as a Sickle cell crisis) in my legs, which was common for me.

I learned to let my professors know that I was registered with the Office of Disability Students Services, and I made copies of my letter directly available to professors if they needed it. This lets professors know that you could need accommodation during your exams. Don't be afraid to speak up with your professors! Let them know that you are aware that there are abuses of the system that might put you at a disadvantage. You need to assert your innocence and let them know that you are not one of those abusers of the system, that you have a legitimate illness and you need appropriate accommodation.

Chapter 10~ Accommodation

For a while in college I did not know that I had Sickle Cell disease, but that did *not* stop Sickle Cell disease from having me. I once had to ask for an extension for an assignment because I had gotten really sick. I remember the Calculus professor saying that I probably had too much alcohol to drink that weekend and that's why I didn't complete my assignment, probably hanging out with "the frat guys". I was so insulted I was silent! There must have been a look of horror on my face, because he quickly realized that he had pegged me wrong, and he started stuttering an apology. I further validated that he was way off by finding my voice to tell him about myself and my ministry on campus. But I should not have even had to do that.

My point? It really helps to have a validated letter from your physician. Teachers are up against very healthy but lazy students trying to "get one over" on their professors because of their own poor discipline with assignments. Professors will think of you this way if you don't legitimize yourself with the right documents.

Chapter 11~ Managing with Coursework

As far as how you manage your time and schedule, be careful not to take very difficult classes during times of the year that are hardest for you, such as during the cold season when Sickle Cell leaves us the most vulnerable. If a crucial class is only offered in the winter, you may want to decide ahead of time to disclose your risk factors for taking classes in the winter. You can then make arrangements either to get an incomplete or take the final exam a week or so later. Even a little extra time might allow you to work with your compromised body to get the work done, depending on how sick you become.

Chapter 11 ~ Managing with Coursework

I was not always well enough to go to class, so I learned by directly studying the text books. Sometimes I was well enough to get together and study with friends. I found those times to be quite valuable-when we actually studied! My time was valuable because I was not operating with the same amounts of free hours as everyone else. So, if you wasted my time and called it studying, you were less likely to see me again. I needed to pass my classes, and there was not enough time to waste.

This reminds me of something I need to share. Sometimes while in classes, I would find myself "snapping out" of what was supposedly just a "wandering mind" episode, or daydreaming. It never affected my overall performance because I always reviewed the required text book chapters before my exams. However, things came to a head when I took an

Ecology class that was entirely based on the lectures of the professor.

I remember being so scared one lecture in particular. When the session was over I had very few notes to show for it. I decided to borrow the notes of a classmate so that I could "fill in" my notes, only to find that I had missed so much it was as if I never attended the lecture! After that point I brought in a tape recorder and recorded my lectures even while present and taking notes, so that I could again "fill in" the gaps. This is the first time that I became aware of how many gaps appeared in my attention span in a lecture only 75 minutes long.

Over the years we found a few things that could have been contributing to this, one of which was my oxygen saturation, or rather desaturations. At first it was hard to diagnose because while sitting and getting my vitals taken, my oxygen saturation was almost always above 97%. But at random times I would stop breathing, and my oxygen levels would fall to as low as 75%, no kidding!

It was also because of these "drifts" during classes that I was finally evaluated one year with a brain MRI, which did in fact show abnormality resulting from chronic sickling in the brain, and damage known as lacunar infarcts. I would have never known that! It was because of this information that I was advised to request extra time for my standardized testing, and any other testing that was particularly time sensitive.

Unfortunately, I did not figure out any of this until years later. We can never assume that we are operating at 100% in our classes. If you suspect there may be challenges in your learning environment, or with your actual processing, err on the side of caution and do not hesitate to sound the alarm. It is always better to do this sooner rather than later.

Chapter 11 ~ Managing with Coursework

Much of the advice I give is based on being in a physical classroom setting, which was my way of schooling. However, now, *you* have the benefit of online schooling as an option. This is a great option for many reasons including the fact that you have more control over your environment and how you learn. However, there may also be issues of concern, like the fact that you will likely have no choice but to study alone. I don't know how this is handled. Also, you would certainly have to be more self- motivated, since there might be less accountability felt remotely. Online courses also tend to move faster, and the workload may be heavier at any given time. Not to mention, studying entirely at home may cause you to have less interpersonal and networking skills that are important assets.

Having said all this, it is a wonderful option for someone with limited mobility, and for people who are self-motivated, all the concerns I mentioned would be a non-issue. It is still worth considering that you can never have too much support. And as it turns out, learning to be supportive of others, and learning to work and build as a team is a crucial part of your education and overall growth. With the birth of some of the recent technology, you can get this almost as well in online schooling as with the traditional school setting.

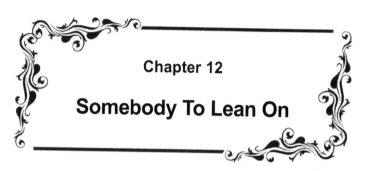

Chapter 12

Somebody To Lean On

I could not have made it through college without the help of my mom and sister. They were amazing. They would team up and my mom would cook many of the Guyanese foods I grew up on and longed for at school. My mom is an excellent cook who loves people by feeding them with her delicious food. She is quite known in our family and social community as being unmatched in her cooking skills. We would all eat, lick our fingers and ask for more!

Whenever I called home to let them know I needed help, and she was able, she got to task. She would cook several dishes, fill each container of food to the brim, and pack them carefully in a bag that my sister would bring to me. It was usually during a time when I was experiencing a Sickle Cell crisis, and was laid up in my bed, and I would call home to let them know what was going on. My sister would gather the food and take a train into the city and arrive while I was in my sick bed. She would sniff the air pungent with body odor and insist that I get up and take a shower. While I was getting cleaned up she would make up my bed with fresh sheets so that I could at least feel human during these dehumanizing episodes of pain. She would do my laundry down the hall in the dormitory. Then after combing my hair and doing anything else that was needed in my room, we would sit and talk and eat.

My mom would call to make sure all went well and that I enjoyed the food. I still remember how happy it made her to hear that I still had a hearty appetite for her cooking. In her mind, I was not eating well on the school's meal plan. She was partially right. Considering that I had a *fully-paid* meal plan, I hardly saw the dining hall when I was sick. On the days when my body was hurting, it felt like a walk across Manhattan to get there.

So, indeed I was grateful for the hearty and familiar meals from my mom's kitchen. That was love, from both my mom and my sister. I felt their love and needed it so much during these times. When I finally graduated from college, I said to my family, "we graduated!" And I meant every word.

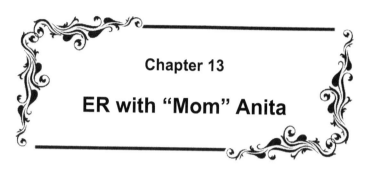

Chapter 13

ER with "Mom" Anita

In my sophomore year at Columbia University, all the students in the campus ministry of our church were given a list of available married couples that we could pick from that volunteered to "adopt" us college kids and watch over us during our schooling, especially during those stressful exam periods and when we could not go home for a holiday. I was excited.

I remembered I made sure to tell my future white parents that my skin was the color of brown sugar! I'm not sure why that was important to me at the time, but it was. Maybe I wanted to give them a heads up to walk away if they so chose. I vaguely remember that they had a super encouraging response especially to that comment, something along the lines of liking brown sugar. It was the start of a beautiful relationship that would span decades.

Most surrogate families concerned themselves with making care packages of food during finals for their college student. My surrogates found themselves rushing to emergency rooms because I was constantly in the hospital, admitted for a transfusion here and infection there. It was way more than they were ever supposed to sign up for, but if they were weary, they never showed it.

I remember once while awaiting admission in a room of the Columbia Presbyterian Emergency department, my "Mom Anita" came bounding in asking to see her "daughter". Now this was a middle-aged woman with the blondest of curls and light brown eyes. So, you can imagine that they were naturally trying to match her with a child of similar description, especially since the love in her heart made her fail to see the problem that would likely ensue without some clarification.

Hearing her voice, I jumped to the rescue of the nurse, who I could hear entering the cubicles of other patients she likely deemed a match, only to be wrong each time. I called out "mom, I'm in here!" "Oh baby! What happened?" She followed my voice and bounded ahead of the nurse to my bedside. The comedy in my head was too much to keep me from smiling as I saw the very confused look on the face of the nurse, having woefully failed in her matchmaking. All while my Mom Anita, clueless of the confusion, expressed her sadness that I was in this awful predicament again. Her love just had no boundaries.

But it proved valuable in another unexpected way. Sickle Cell disease is unfortunately an illness where patients are easily labeled as drug seekers because of the amount and intensity of pain associated with a Sickle Cell crisis. It is a cruel and insulting journey of pain that often left me with heightened emotions spewing in every direction. I was mad that it was happening again, sad that it was costing me so much of my life even as I was trying to complete my pre-medical studies in the hopes of going to medical school. I was always afraid that the doctors and nurses I encountered would not understand Sickle Cell disease and that these could be my last days. I was embarrassed that someone would even think this was an act just to get IV drugs, as though I had nothing better to do with my life!

At such a time, having a Caucasian mom as an advocate seemed to legitimize my emergency room experience. This is so very hard to admit, because for a long time, I was not sure if it was all in my head or truly happening. It was so subtle! But nurses seemed to become kinder to me, more patient even. And I was suddenly able to relax and explain my situation with more clarity, address my expectations of the visit or admission, and settle down to a calmer hospital visit even when things did not go my way.

To be sure, it was not always the case that I felt dismissed or pre-judged. I had experienced a great many doctors who were friendly to me and encouraged me that it was safe to advocate for my needs and say what medicine worked and how much. But I had received more than my share of doctors who were insensitive and unkind. This is an unfortunate narrative of people with Sickle Cell disease. For anyone who has significant pain that requires intervention and help from medical professionals, you will hear this familiar complaint of their treatment. When you hear it enough times even from people you know to be good-natured, you realize that there must be some element of truth to it.

Unfortunately, the biggest complaints that patients have were legitimized years later as a practicing physician, when healthcare providers complained to me about the hang-ups they had with Sickle Cell patients. I remember one nurse talking to a pharmacist on the floor. She said, "you know what makes me mad, when I see the patient's head bobbing, and they are almost passed out from the pain medicine, and yet they're still asking for more! Now tell me that is not drug-seeking behavior!"

I had to explain to them both that there is a big difference between pain control and sedation. Many of the medications given, for every 1 point of pain control let's say, had 3 points for sedation. When you doubled a tiny quantity, there was now

2 points for pain control, but *6* points for sedation! Sadly, these healthcare providers were seeing sedation and equating it with pain control, and labeling patients as drug-seekers because of heavy sedation. Often, as I experienced myself, my pain was intense enough to awaken me from deep sleep, crying out for relief. And with good reason. Sickle Cell pain has been likened to end stage cancer pain, which is why it is treated with the same medications. I just wish we were always given the same amount of dignity as we take those medications. We are traumatized by the disease and further traumatized by being humiliated while asking for help.

But back there with Mom Anita during my college years, having her around made me feel like no one would ignore my plea for help. I was young, and often felt vulnerable, but with her I knew someone was watching out for me. No matter what happened, I was going to be okay. The world was as it should be, or as close to it as possible.

As silly as this may seem, the option to go from feeling harassed and helpless to feeling some sense of control is a powerful one. And whether the dangers were real or imagined, I am sure that my sudden feeling of peace and possibility of good outcome affected my perception of pain and my ability to cope with each Sickle Cell battle in front of me. Her kindness was a cushion upon which I could fall when life itself felt like it had punched me out.

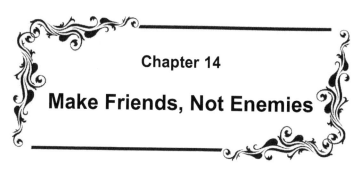

Chapter 14

Make Friends, Not Enemies

I had just come back from doing one of my blood exchange transfusions where 3 to 5 units of blood- depending on the week- was given to me after my own red blood cells were harvested, isolated in an Electrophoresis Machine, and thrown away in a red hazard trash bag. I came back tired but hopeful knowing that in a day or so, my new red blood cells would kick in and I would be like superwoman or the Energizer Bunny with the nonstop battery. And I happened to have made it to class that day, only to realize that Dr. C, my biology professor, was teaching about Sickle Cell Disease! All was going well until, in order to be original and keep the class engaged he said (of Sickle Cell patients), "…and they usually kick the bucket by age 20 years old".

At first, I thought I was dreaming. Then, I was livid. I was 20, and for darn sure I was planning on seeing 21, and I did not need his song playing in my brain. So, after class that day I marched up to him, took a deep breath, barely contained, and greeted him. I let him know that I was Simone Eastman (my maiden name), a student in his class, who after coming back from my life-giving exchange transfusion had to sit there while he told me and the rest of the class that I was pretty much going to die by the age of 20! I don't much remember what else I said except that I do remember straining back the tears as I told him that I had Sickle Cell disease, that I was 20 years old, and that I intended with every fiber in me to beat those odds!

I thought he would be defensive. I thought he would shut me down and make excuses and point to the fact that the textbooks supported him. Instead he looked intrigued, happy even, and stretched out his hand to shake mine. I remember that like it was yesterday. In essence he told me that he was very proud that I had stepped forward to defend myself, that he was very pleased to meet someone with Sickle Cell disease in his biology class, and apologized for the way he said what he said in the class, honestly admitting that he would have never thought that someone with Sickle Cell disease was sitting in his classroom.

I could have been so ticked off that I did not see the possibility of friendship. I could have rejected the handshake. But in that moment, I decided I wanted a friend. And just like that we were friends. He asked me not to be a stranger and said he would not be one either. He said hello whenever he saw me, and from time to time I dropped by his office for one biology-related thing or another.

Chapter 14 ~ Make Friends, Not Enemies

Funny enough befriending my professor made me feel like it was OK to ask questions about my class, when I should've felt that to begin with. Which brings me to the point that you should always go and say hello and break the ice with your professors because that small step opens up your confidence in a way that allows you to get all the possible help that you need for your classes and coursework. That was not the original intention, but it certainly became a wonderful consequence.

I remember when I suddenly had to leave New York, he became instrumental in pairing me up with a professor at UCLA to complete my studies. It was winter of 1993 and I had one more class to complete and one exam to be proctored. But that winter in New York triggered an urgent move. It was incredibly cold, and I was hospitalized at Columbia-Presbyterian for a Sickle Cell crisis while my dear friend Anna Stacey was hospitalized at another hospital in Manhattan. To make a long story short, I made it out of the hospital, but my kindred spirit did not. Instead her systems crashed, overwhelmed by the sickling in her body. I made it to her bedside and spoke into her ear letting her know that it was OK to let go if it was too much, if it was too painful, and promised her that I would make it through medical school for the both of us, that I would see to it that I finished and became a doctor like we promised each other we would be.

But that meant finishing my coursework, and New York was proving to be too cold for that. It was proving to be incompatible with life if you ask me. The only option was to run. With the help of my church family we were able to contact a family in Los Angeles who included me in a household so that I could be anchored there. Dr. C was instrumental in helping me connect with a professor at UCLA who would be the point person for receiving my completed coursework, as well as proctoring my final departmental exam. I also remember him trying to gently coax me into applying to UCLA for medical school. I never told him this, but I was so thankful to him for believing in me that I would be able to complete my mission. In the years to come as I found out what it really took to complete medical school, I have looked back on our friendship and on his mentoring. As I remember his vote of confidence, I have been grateful for whatever brief moment it was that he was in my life. He played more of a significant role than he probably ever imagined.

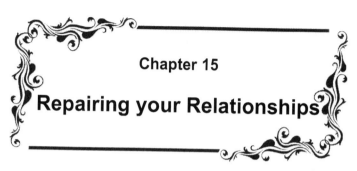

Chapter 15

Repairing your Relationships

My people in the struggle, I need to share something with you regarding your friendships. Most of us, by the time we are adults, have a very thinned out support system. We have been sick, all our lives, and have had to reach out for a helping hand many, many times. Some of us have still managed to continue with a pretty healthy support system around us, even into our 30s and 40s. But many have a hard time with a waning fan base as we grow older, and here is why.

Just by the nature of what has happened to us, we have become takers. We did not mean it and did not assume this position on purpose;

it was gifted to us along with the unpredictable and life-threatening nature of this painful illness. It happened when we least expected it, at very inconvenient times to the people we love.

The state of chaos we exist in is usually ok for occasional disasters, but living like this week after week, year after year becomes exhausting. Lovely, well-meaning people who start out willing to help us eventually begin to feel used up in the process, which is no fault of ours by the way. However, if we do not take some time to reverse the damage our relationships have suffered, these people can suffer burnout slowly and over time, leaving us to fend for ourselves. We may never be able to repay them, but you will need to encourage them on some level.

Now all encouragements are not equal- we need to love up on them in a way best received by each individual supporter. What do I mean by this? The year I read about "The Five Love Languages" by Gary Chapman was a year of such clarity for me. It finally helped me understand why some people, despite my best efforts to exercise the biblical principle of loving people, did not feel like their love and support of me was reciprocated. However, after reading this book, a book I highly recommend by the way, I understood why this was happening. I became intentional about loving my friends in the way they understood and best received love. The response was amazing! I certainly felt like and saw that I was meeting the needs of these precious people. Many of them had poured their own lives into mine during times when I was sick and needed it most. And with deep gratitude, I wanted to make sure they were adequately rejuvenated from the process of helping me.

I knew that I was on the right track when people left their healthy, physically fit friends who could do all manner of social things with them, and came to hang out with me, with my portable oxygen wearing, cane carrying limping self! And they were quite content to sit on my couch, or in some cases by my bedside, and chat away like we were at our favorite restaurant! I went from a time in my life where people hardly remembered when I was sick and dropped out of sight, to people wanting to include me in their lives. People came to visit me in the hospital and said to me, "good, now I get to have you all to myself, at least until the next person walks in".

People told me that when they hear that I'm home recuperating they "jump at the chance to hang out" because otherwise I'm "always surrounded by people". I have friends that will come and take me to an art show in the park even though they have to push me in my wheelchair. Even when I feel awkward about them having to do such strenuous activity, they will stand there and talk me into it and exclaim joyfully when I finally agree to go. People call or text to see if I need anything, and gladly bring things I randomly request even when I'm not sick and in need.

I cannot keep people out of my house! While some of this is without a doubt good will from the Christian hearts of my friends, I believe that loving people intentionally and individually helps their hearts and influences their actions. It was these same people who acted differently after being loved "in their language". While it still takes me by surprise at times, the truth is that loving people this way will always yield fruit. It is a biblical principle.

I really would suggest you do the same for your own relationships. During random times of sitting with your friends and loved ones, ask them what makes them feel loved and special, and LISTEN to what they say. My suggestion would be to start with the relationships you feel like you are struggling with; the ones that seem to need the most TLC. If you do this enough, you will hear the similarities and differences of your supporters in terms of what makes them feel loved. Make a mental note of what they are telling you. Feel free to even jot it down someplace reliable, like in your phone book under their name. Whatever it takes, remember it. Whenever you want to encourage them, use this information to be specific, catering to their individual needs.

By the way, you should be looking at all your friends and how to love them long before you ever need anything from them. Truthfully the hope is that a need never arises! This is not about what you can get from people. This is your intentional attempt to love these people in your world the best way you know how.

One other thing I will say about this. I have found that you do not have to do much to make people feel loved. Often, it's the thought or the effort that counts. You may not be able to buy an elaborate present. However, taking the time to make a handmade card or collage, anything that shows effort, goes a long way. Anything that reflects that it was done specifically with them in mind versus a generic gift is highly encouraging. The fact that you who are physically disabled and struggling has made such an effort to encourage them goes an incredibly long way, more than you know!

Another building block of great friendships is to give encouragement. Give it freely and often. I do not mean that you should lie, but in order to do this correctly, you will need to pay close attention to the positive things you hear and see in people. It has always been there. No one is all good or all bad. But sometimes you do have to train your eyes and ears to see the good in people. Most importantly, give this encouragement publicly! It is the closest thing to having the whole room cheering for that person when you give a compliment to them and everyone around them hears and agrees with the compliment as well.

Another simple way to encourage that is sure to uplift the people who support you often is to tell them when things are going well, or when you are feeling better. People who love you will be around you often when things are falling apart. If all they think of when they see you is heartache, this will be challenging. You really need to remember to tell them every positive thing that happens. Celebrate that your pain flare calmed down and you feel "almost normal" today. Share with them when your blood test comes back with positive results. Tell them when you are able to have a particularly productive day, even if it took unconventional means to accomplish your goals.

Lastly, thank your friends profusely, often, and publicly as well. This is especially the case if they have in some way communicated to you that it took a lot to do whatever they did for you. Please be sincere here, because people can very often tell if you are not, and you stand a chance of causing that friendship harm. Working on giving genuine thanks is a great way to reflect on all you have been given and you are grateful for.

You will have to study each friend to know if they are one of a few people that may become uncomfortable by these gestures. By and large most people yearn to have positive attention. For those whose love language is to be praised, this will strengthen them immensely!

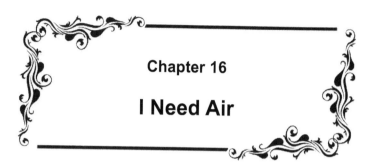

Chapter 16

I Need Air

One of the things that was hard for me was to admit that I needed assistance in basic things like walking from a building to the parking lot. But when I finally fessed up and got the help, I saved so much energy! I had so much left to make it through the day that I realized very quickly it was worth it. But getting to this point of clarity did not come easy.

The first thing I realized was that with each episode of sickling, I was experiencing shortness of breath progressively. I could not figure out whether the symptoms were a result of the previous damages to my lung tissue or the frequent pneumonias I kept having, or from ongoing sickling. Whatever it was, I was huffing as I walked and panting as I talked. It was becoming harder to walk long distances, and I was tired walking any significant distance.

With great reluctance I went to my pulmonologist and asked if I could have a disability placard to park closer to buildings. He looked at me in shock and said, "I thought you already had one of those just for your Sickle Cell!" So, this kind man had already figured that considering the extreme fatigue Sickle Cell brings, I had already received a permanent parking placard from my primary care physician or at least my hematologist. Not only did I not have one, but I waited until I was very out of breath before feeling comfortable enough asking for one!

We can be quite cruel to ourselves when we have a chronic invisible illness, in part because we may look normal and have a hard time explaining to people why we have the needs we do. And to be sure it is a little difficult if you are not using any assistive devices as you walk to disability parking, because people are so brainwashed into thinking only visibly disabled people need those accommodations! They look at you strangely, and being so young, I got all the scornful looks, as though I was not entitled to the placard I was using.

But the one thing that made me not care about the scornful looks and stares was the fact that I felt significantly better parking closer and saving energy. The difference was obvious! There had been times when I would walk to my car and by the time I got there I would feel too tired to drive, and somewhat spacey, so I would sit there for a while. Those times were pretty much cut in half if not more simply by parking closer with the aid of a placard.

Chapter 16 ~ I Need Air

I decided to test my oxygen levels to see if I could find anything that would explain to me why I would feel the way I did when walking for even one block. And I was astonished with what I found! Every time I had a clinic visit, my oxygen levels were always between 97 and 100% as I sat there calmly while they took my vitals. I assumed that this therefore was the status quo for my body, that I was functioning with oxygen saturations above 97% at most times. Not so my friend!

A friend of mine who was curious about my symptoms decided to get me a pulse oximeter. Now this was before we had Amazon and could order nifty little devices like a finger oximeter. Instead, this sucker looked like a laptop. It had its own bag to tote around, with wired probes that wrapped around my finger, and connected to the laptop device via a long cord. Let's just say you saw me coming!

Chapter 16 ~ I Need Air

But I did not care! I wanted some answers too, and I was so grateful to my friend for being able to track down something like this that I could use. As I started using it, I started noticing that at rest my oxygen saturations were consistently above 97% for the most part. Then for seconds at a time, it would trend downward to the mid to high 80s and bounce right back up again.

Okay... so my oxygen dropped sometimes at rest, but only for seconds at a time. No big deal, right? Well not if that was all. I decided to "suit up" with my probe and bag and walk longer distances, and sure enough my oxygen saturation would drop mid to high 70s and remain that way even after I stopped walking! Now that's more than seconds! And by the time I reached the parking lot, I was breathing heavily. I took notes of each drop, and how far it was that I walked to reflect these numbers. It was not far at all.

Chapter 16 ~ I Need Air

What was more devastating was climbing stairs! I plummeted quickly and stayed desaturated longer, with a slow rebound to normal that was about 4-5 minutes duration. Because of the low levels I was seeing, I would stop walking for a little while after climbing the stairs before continuing down the hallway of whichever floor I had climbed to. But I shuddered to think of what my poor body endured when I was not aware, when I continued trudging down the hall after climbing stairs, not knowing how low my oxygen had gotten just by climbing the stairs! My body was enduring a lot, and no one noticed.

I finally took these finding to my Pulmonologist at the time, a wonderful doctor I refer to as Dr. John who worked with the attending physician. By the end of my visit I was scheduled for a pulmonary function test, and another evaluation known as a Six-Minute Walk Test. I did not know it then, but those tests would forever change my life as I knew it.

Chapter 16 ~ I Need Air

I turned myself in for a pulmonary function test and a Six-Minute Walk Test both of which confirmed that I was desaturating, and my oxygen was indeed falling to the mid-70s, when it should have been above 89%. A result of 89% saturation or below is the point at which you are required to wear supplemental oxygen. The reason for this is that under 89% saturation there is a sharp fall in the oxygenation of your tissues, putting your brain and the rest of your body at risk for irreversible brain and organ damage.

No wonder I was feeling so crappy after walking through the parking lot to my car. By the time I reached my car I was probably starving my whole body of oxygen! It certainly explained why I felt too tired to even drive. Once I was given the portable supplemental oxygen, a couple of things became obvious. The first is that I was *not* breathless everywhere. I no longer walked around huffing and panting while I spoke. And I made it to my car without feeling spacey or needing to take five minutes before driving.

But there was another curious thing that happened. Because I now had a portable oxygen unit with a nasal cannula(tubing) in my nose - a visible sign of a handicap- people left me alone. In fact, most people smiled or nodded hello as I approached my car. Suddenly I had some sort of "permission" to use the disabled parking, as though my condition was a new manifestation. My symptoms had been there all along, and ironically, I was much doing worse back then for *not* having the portable oxygen.

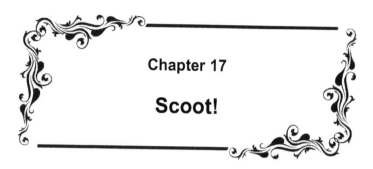

Chapter 17

Scoot!

Along the way I discovered other things that minimized my exertion. Basically, I made my life easy by using whatever I could. This time it was the scooters in the stores. I started riding scooters around in supermarkets and any store that carried them. My reason for doing this was simple. I had started to recognize patterns. I would come home very tired after a shopping trip and simply fall apart at home. My legs ached, and my arms. My chest and mid back would ache. It would take me a minimum of two days- and usually more- just to bounce back from that pain and fatigue.

Chapter 17 ~ Scoot!

I started hating shopping, for anything! It did not matter whether it was for my favorite foods at specialty stores or needing to upgrade my wardrobe or buying a gift for someone. I stopped going to the store and asked my family or friends to get something for me wherever and whenever they were going.

Now, I'm sure you've been in a position where you sent someone to the store with your hard-earned money to buy something, and someway somehow, they get it so very wrong! You're so frustrated because they are not enthusiastic to return to the store just to return or exchange one item. Then to add insult to injury they tell you they were not planning on returning to that store in a while. All you could do is take the receipt and the bought item and hope you might be able to take it back yourself. *That* was the reason I had to create a Plan B.

Chapter 17 ~ Scoot!

I started using scooters around the stores before there was any visible evidence of my disease, like my portable oxygen or the cane I use today. And even then, I did not care who was staring. I was shedding my pride and figuring out that the only way to get what I wanted was to do it myself by any ethical means necessary. And the scooter was necessary, just like the placard was too. Like before, it was quite interesting watching people stare at me trying to figure out why a very young well-dressed African-American woman with no visible handicap would need to ride around in a scooter. Nonetheless I persisted each time and boldly went to the place in every store where the scooters were, climbed in and zoomed away. I could speed up my shopping, lessen the wear and tear on my body, and recuperate for a few hours, not "resurrect" days later.

Chapter 17 ~ Scoot!

And as the years passed and I got to wearing portable oxygen, it was even nicer to have a place to rest that heavy tank of oxygen. It was nice not to have to haul that around the store. Years later, after 5 hip-replacement surgeries, walking became even more difficult for me. I did indeed have to lessen my visits to the supermarkets and department stores. But scooters were still my friends when I did go. And they still are today.

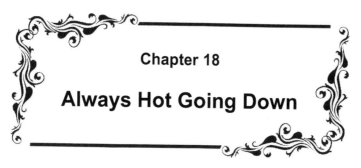

Chapter 18

Always Hot Going Down

This one I discovered by accident. I was desperate to go to a conference which was being held at a hotel with heavily air-conditioned rooms, which has always been my nemesis. It's the upset of walking into the supermarket for only a few minutes, and walking out with a Sickle Cell crisis triggered, simply because the store was too cold for me. And sometimes it did not seem to matter that you bundled yourself up before going into the store. The moment you got out, you knew that all your fancy layered dressing was for naught. I carried a thick jacket wherever I went. In fact, I kept several jackets and coats in the trunk of my car. I could never underestimate the power of walking from a sunny outside to a highly air-conditioned building. And I have paid dearly for not heeding to those temperature transition points.

So, I took a heating pad with me, and had the idea to take my thermos with hot water so that I could drink it in the cold room. And don't you know once I started drinking the hot water in the room, I felt like a normal human being for the rest of the day and even into the next day, which was more than I could ever ask for operating in all of these air-conditioned facilities.

I decided to take my new buffer to church, a place where I would always get cold. It did not help that many people had post-menopausal hot flashes and wanted a nice cool building. I was clearly outnumbered! I would dress up like I was taking off for the north pole, so much so that my friend Millie exclaimed one day "my gosh, *looking* at you makes me feel hot!" Yet, I would still experience such discomfort! I'd have to walk out of the service and just wait for the people to start filtering outside to have any chance of fellowship with them. I usually waited outside in my car.

But once I started taking my thermos to church with me, it was a different ball game altogether. I was able to stay in the service and continue right to the end. My friends, happy to see that something was working, would happily refill my cup with hot water from the church kitchen. They took turns keeping a steady supply of hot water coming for me to drink.

Now there are times when it doesn't work and for the life of me I don't know why. But for the most part my episodes in the cold have been greatly alleviated by sipping on hot water. When the normal body is trying to conserve heat in a cold place, the vessels will constrict (tighten, narrow) to retain the body's heat, to protect the body from becoming too cold. For our bodies with Sickle Cell Disease however, sudden vasoconstriction in the cold is not nice. Narrowing those vessels to prevent heat from escaping can also cause increased obstruction of the flow of blood, robbing tissues of oxygen which can lead to damage, or death, of those tissues. So, we find ourselves hurting badly during these times.

Drinking hot water on a cold day can fool the body into thinking that you are overheating, causing the vessels to dilate instead of constricting. In doing so, we keep the blood vessels open, decreasing the chances of blockage that would normally come. We have to drink hot liquids continuously during this time to keep the body in an overheated state with dilated vessels so that we reduce the tendency for blockage and pain. And hey! If you're going to drink hot water all the time, you might as well add some lemon into it and get great digestion, cleansing of the gallbladder, and if you need it- some weight loss too!

PART III

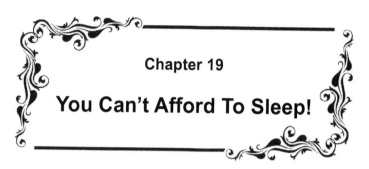

Chapter 19

You Can't Afford To Sleep!

I have shared quite a bit of things to help you find incentive for navigating your way to better education and empowerment in general. I know that it is not the easiest thing to leave the life you have known, even if it is broken, and reach out for something better. And I'm sure many of you, despite me letting you in on my humble beginnings, will likely think that there was some exception that made me excel, and that is somehow off limits to you. *Not* true!

As one of two children from a single parent family who grew up in a developing country like Guyana, struggling to make ends meet, I can tell you that initially my biggest motivator to do better was ending poverty. I liked the idea of having meals regularly, and I wanted to have enough to eat for a change. As I grew into adulthood my reasons changed, but the ability to take care of my health and beat the statistics for Sickle Cell disease survival was never far from my mind. I did not just want life, but a better quality of life. I wanted to be a Sickle Cell thriver, not just a survivor!

When I was younger I thought that as long as I had health insurance, my health needs were covered. This could not be further from the truth! I found that the nutrition and supplements and therapies that showed the most promise for Sickle Cell disease were hardly ever covered by health insurance. Honestly this is also the case for many chronic diseases. It became obvious after a while that I would have to *wake up* and get educated, get informed and get going.

I also reminded myself that it was not just about me. My loved ones feel the consequences of every decision I make, good or bad. Also, being a follower of God reminds me that I cannot hide out because of my diagnosis with Sickle Cell disease. God still expects me to do the very best with what he has given me, even if I only had one talent. He wants to use me right where I am. He may not expect the same thing of me that He does of others, but He expects my best! And He knows what my best is. These days I pray, ask for guidance, and go forth giving it my best, whatever that looks like on any given day. And when tomorrow comes, I will try again.

There is truly nothing like education. Regardless of your background and where you start, once you have been educated, and your eyes have been opened, no human being can take that away from you. On your worst day, as long as you are conscious and without brain injury, you will always have the knowledge you obtain as you journey through your life. And you can look yourself in the mirror and be proud that your DNA defined you in a positive way. Believe me when I say that your knowledge has the potential for you to be the greatest of help to yourself and to many *if* you use it!

Let me be the first to say that I don't intend for you to join the rest of the world in an office cubicle with a 9 to 5 job. I can't do that and honestly many people *without* physical limitations desire to be far away from that as possible. But when you are educated, oh my! Your physical environment may not have changed and yet suddenly you are seeing the world in a very new and different way. You speak with people differently, and your language changes so remarkably that you are able to use your words in a powerful way.

Chapter 19 ~ You Can't Afford To Sleep!

What comes out of your mouth as a result of being enlightened lets people know they are messing with the wrong person and need to adjust themselves. Someone who may have known you all their life will realize that you have been awakened and empowered. And because of this transformation, you are now able to use your acquired tools to influence the hearts and minds of the people around you. All because you took a chance, and you chose to dream big, and grow!

There are so many careers that need your beautiful brain without needing so much of your physical body. With the birth of online business and commerce, the possibilities are endless for you. I wish I had this technology starting out, truly. It is simply a matter of going for what you love and thinking outside of the box if what you want to do does not currently exist. Every business, every lucrative idea that exists today had to be started by someone. Why not you? You may have to create your own lane, but create away my kindred spirit, create! The good thing about these options is that if you lay the foundation early enough and start on whatever you want to do, when the time comes where you are too physically compromised to do much, you will be able to sit back and reap from what you have already planted. This principle by the way applies in all areas, whether it be residual income or investing in relationships and friendships early so that when hard times come you know where to turn.

Even today as I face more challenges from aging with Sickle Cell disease that has made me slow down, I'm still discovering new and unconventional ways to use my education. Right now, for example, I'm writing this book! I can still give general medical input, or review some medical records for a friend, just to help people in general who may not have the means to see a physician.

For people who help me take care of my health, I make sure to use any number of my abilities to bless them in some way as a token of my appreciation. Thankfully, I am still able to have some amount of positive impact in general. In looking at all I have already been able to do, I consider myself very fortunate.

I realize that because I was diagnosed relatively late, and I had significant complications early in life that were not properly treated, my course may be different from yours. I'm certainly hoping that with whatever guidance I can provide, you will be able to soar, and set yourself up in a way that allows you some enjoyment of life and betterment of your health.

Chapter 19 ~ You Can't Afford To Sleep!

The more you embrace education, the more it opens your eyes to what is available, what your needs are, and how best to advocate for yourself, and even others.

With all the technology you now have at your fingertips, you really have a good shot of having a user-friendly way to a better life. I can only imagine how much easier it would have been to go to school via online courses. These days it is a perfectly acceptable alternative. Back when I was going through college, it did not even exist. There would have been so much more flexibility in using this option, although I can easily see that accommodation would have to be made for online schooling as well.

Unlike me who had to stumble along and fall many times while creating a way for myself, you have the benefit of knowing what to do before you start. Please do not take this for granted. My greatest joy would be to see you take my mistakes and learn from them. I wish I had known to register with the Office for Disability Students Services on campus, but unfortunately, I did not know. I did not even know to ask! It caused great heartache in my transition back to school.

I remember leaving an exam early because it was too cold in the exam room and I could feel my body starting to ache and knew that this could lead to an emergency room visit and possible hospitalization if I didn't act quickly. It became impossible to concentrate because my legs were hanging for over two hours and throbbed so much that the only thing I was concentrating on was how to make it stop. Unfortunately, at first, I did not know to ask for help. After several lesser performances on exams from different classes because of Sickle Cell related difficulties in the test taking environment, I started becoming truly alarmed that my future in medicine would be thwarted. I started asking advice on what to do. I was finally told that there was an Office for Disability Students Services on campus that could advocate for me, and likely all I needed was a letter from my doctor. Can you imagine me correcting the situation and watching my grades go right back up? I could not believe it.

At first, I felt very insecure that I needed these accommodations because of my life-threatening diagnosis. But I remember an advisor explaining to me that if I did not know the subject material, if I had not studied and prepared, no amount of accommodation would suddenly cause me to know that material and excel on an exam. She reassured me that instead of me having to run a race with my legs tied while everyone was running with their legs untied, we were finding a way to level the playing field. I'm trying to level *your* playing field!

Lastly, I'm so glad that I learned to recognize my strengths and use them as leverage for things I needed. It was so hard on my self-esteem feeling like I had nothing to offer anyone, and yet I was in constant need of help. Thinking of yourself as bringing something to the table allows you to feel more like you are in a partnership and less like a charity case. This is important because even when people try to reassure us that we are not a burden, we can often still feel that way.

Daring to dream of higher education with your diagnosis of Sickle Cell disease and chronic pain can seem overwhelming. However, I believe you can see now why getting an education is well worth it. Furthermore, many of the ways to navigate to your goal that I have shared with you can ease your strain and make your dreams a reality. With all this being the case, it would be truly a waste to not pursue an education in something that would elevate your quality of life. And the time is here. It is now. And it is yours for the taking, one careful step at a time.

No man is an island however, and your relationships will be key in you being able to make this journey. As I mentioned a while back, learning to be there for people was not always my strength. As I look back it is easy to see how I made life more difficult for myself in the times when I did not nurture my relationships, and I likely caused some of them to experience burnout. Learn from this! Take the time to put the work in to nourish and protect your relationships, it will be well worth your investment.

This is your journey; learn to use whatever (legal and ethical) means is necessary to get there! Don't worry much about how you are looking in the moment. Concentrate on maximizing your energy and taking care of yourself as best you can along the way, so that you can finish the journey. As I also mentioned earlier in the book, using a scooter while food shopping is better than walking around and looking cute and fitting in when you know full well you will pay for it later. You don't have time for extra pain when you are pursuing your dream of "becoming".

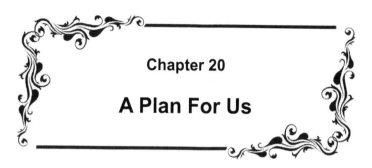

Chapter 20

A Plan For Us

The fact that you are reading this book right now is no accident. It was meant for you, for such a time as this. I was sent as a guide to somehow use what I am blessed with, to hopefully help you use what you are blessed with.

You have been given much. Don't just look at the circumstances. Look at what it can display, you! The manger displayed Jesus! Your DNA is simply your backdrop that will enhance the amazing work that you will do. It will undoubtedly inspire many who will watch as you shine in your circumstances.

Chapter 20 ~ A Plan For Us

I recently heard someone say about writers that our message may be the key to someone else's future. That statement resonated with me, because this book was given to me to write years ago. At that time, I was barely able to balance my life as a Christian, a wife, a daughter, a sister, and a practicing Family Medicine doctor battling Sickle Cell disease. I felt spread thin! However, of those titles and roles I held, the only negotiable one was a doctor. Yet, as crazy as health care was becoming, and as disillusioned as I felt, and as much as the physical exertion was impacting my Sickle Cell affected body, I did not know how to walk away. I loved what I did very much. I loved my patients and treated them like my own family, and my yearly office evaluations wherever I worked consistently reflected this.

While recuperating from back to back fourth and fifth hip surgery of my left hip, I received a call from a friend. She said "Simone this is going to sound quite weird, but I've been avoiding calling you for some time now, because I have a message for you, but I don't know how to give you. But God wants you to stop working Simone. He says He wants to take better care of His baby girl, and He promises that you will not have to worry about your needs; He will take care of you."

At this point I was still technically on medical leave, and my employers at Orlando Health had been gracious enough to hold my position this whole time. I got monthly updates about how much my patients missed me, and I got manila envelopes in my mailbox containing the get-well cards mailed to me as my office staff forwarded the well wishes of patients who were eager for my return.

My mind quickly thought about all of this and returned to the phone conversation with my friend,

Tencha. I thanked her for being brave enough to deliver the message. I could only imagine the emotional roller coaster a man or woman of faith goes through when saddled with such a life changing message to deliver. It's not easy to tell a physician, who has trained most of their adult life in the medical field that they should just stop. And do nothing! Not start a ministry, not be a missionary, not change careers. Just STOP. You had to be pretty confident that this was a divinely sent message to be so bold!

That delivered message kept me up for several nights straight. Wow, it would be so nice to finally take care of this body that seems to be crashing and burning under my nose. And what a relief not having to practice my integrative medicine in secret. I hated having to whisper to my patients about natural options for their ailments. Many were clearly wanting this holistic alternative, but they couldn't find doctors that would help, because many of them feared punishment and harm to their licenses. But stop working? Was this the answer? And was this really from God?

Three weeks later, another friend, one with Sickle Cell disease that knew me since my college days called me. HE had a message! And yep-you guessed it!

"Simone God wants you to stop the work you are doing right now and take care of yourself." I cannot remember my exact words, but I must have voiced some fear regarding how I would take care of myself financially. And I will never forget what he said to me. He said, "Simone if you trust God, He will take care of you and you will be provided for better than when you were working as a doctor." I will never forget that promise.

I made up my mind to leave the job. My health was not bouncing back, and I knew I was forcing the issue. I spoke with my husband and was at peace. And sure enough, as if to remove any temptation to renege on my decision, very soon after I was contacted by my employers who (understandably) could no longer hold my job, and so they offered me a severance package instead. It was only a few months later that I was told, after extensive testing, that my lung function had relapsed. I would be returning to portable oxygen after three years of reprieve. Looking back on how things unfolded, it seems like I was being prepared for this news.

I have taken the past few years for the much-needed time to rest and recuperate from all of the unusually hard work it took to get a body with Sickle Cell disease through college, medical school, residency and a career in Family Medicine. Some of that time I seriously questioned God about where we were going. I was certain at one point that I had been taken out of the game and benched, forced to look while the world played on. It was a time of wandering in the spiritual desert for me. I asked all the hard and frightening questions, about whether He still had plans to prosper me and not harm me, and when or if I would rise again. What I learned in the end was that this was preparation. It was for me and for you. For me, it was a time of rest and reflection, and later reinvention and redirection to something powerful-Sickle Cell Advocacy, and advocacy for the chronically pained.

But it was for you as well! It was for me to soon afterwards knock on the door of your life and ask the question: "Hey! You! What are you doing in there?" If the answer is "I'm living my dream. And I'm happy I make a difference", then fantabulous! If it is not however, and you have not figured out how to start living that life of purpose starting from right where you are, then this will not be the end of this conversation.

Chapter 20 ~ A Plan For Us

I must ask you to consider that you, with your Sickle Cell disease, can serve a great purpose. And while it is not an easy task to be sure, you were not meant to be just a survivor. Right now, I ask that you stop, grab a pen and a piece of paper, and write this declaration: "I'm a Sickle Cell Thriver, *not* just a survivor!" To survive is to remain alive where others have died. You don't have to do much more than that. But YOU, you are productive and confident of a great life ahead of you, and ready to follow your dreams. You will have a legacy because you will choose to live and laugh and love the best way you know how. You *are* a thriver! Copy the words on that paper and post it all around you to remind you of this fact: "I'm a Sickle Cell Thriver, *not* just a survivor!"

If you are willing to take a deep breath and ask yourself two exciting questions, you will go quite far! It is said that the journey of a thousand miles begins with a single step. The first of the two questions is, "What would I want to be and do if I did not have Sickle Cell disease?" I want you to pause and allow yourself to dream of two or three things you would be quite happy doing.

Now the next question; "What if I could be and do what I wanted anyway, *with* Sickle Cell disease?" Hold on! This is a reasonable question to entertain. What if you could custom design your way through whatever education was needed to get at least one of those three things you wanted? And what if you could get help? Would you be willing? Because if you are, then your very next step is to write down the first move you can make towards this and choose a deadline of when you will call yourself to action on this move. And there you go! The first step of your journey begins! Congratulations on fighting for you!!!

Chapter 20 ~ A Plan For Us

As I move on to my autobiography, "Come Fly with Me", I wish you the very best that life has to offer. You have so many good things ahead of you! And so do I! Please, look out for my new book. It should be an interesting read, and more for a general audience. If at any point you feel like you are losing your way or need a sounding board for your many amazing ideas, drop me a line and let's make some magic happen!

Made in the USA
Lexington, KY
28 November 2018